THE
MAKER'S
DIET

TRANSFORMATION

JOURNAL

THE
MAKER'S
DIET

TRANSFORMATION

JORDAN RUBIN

DESTINY IMAGE® PUBLISHERS, INC.

P.O. Box 310, Shippensburg, PA 17257-0310

"Promoting Inspired Lives."

This book and all other Destiny Image, Revival Press, MercyPlace, Fresh Bread, Destiny Image Fiction, and Treasure House books are available at Christian bookstores and distributors worldwide.

For a U.S. bookstore nearest you, call 1-800-722-6774.

For more information on foreign distributors, call 717-532-3040.

Reach us on the Internet: www.destinyimage.com.

ISBN 13 TP: 978-0-7684-0370-1

For Worldwide Distribution, Printed in the U.S.A.

1 2 3 4 5 6 7 8 / 17 16 15 14

INTRODUCTION

NOTE FROM JORDAN ABOUT THE UPCOMING TEN-DAY EXPERIENCE.

Get ready. This ten-day transformation experience is so much more than a fast—it is the beginning of a whole new way of doing life!

To see things you have never seen, you must be willing to do some things that, perhaps, you have never done. This is why we have brought you the *Transformation* curriculum. I am convinced that God wants to do things in you that are truly supernatural and revolutionary. He wants to release breakthrough in every area of your life, so that ultimately you go from a person in need of breakthrough to someone who becomes an *agent of breakthrough* to a broken world.

This is what I want to invest into the body of Christ in this incredible season. The church needs a generation of Daniels, willing to be extraordinary in the spheres of influence God has assigned them. Daniel did not just fast for a season and then go back to "normal" life. Rather, Daniel lived a "normal" that we should aspire to today. The result? Wisdom. Protection. Divine favor. Remarkable insight. And perhaps most significantly, time after time, Daniel watched the kings of a godless Babylon acknowledge the Lord as the One True God.

What was the secret to Daniel's spiritual success? He recognized a key that opened doors that cannot be opened by anything else: *Fasting*.

Is this not the fast that I have chosen: to loose the bonds of wick-edness, to undo the heavy burdens, to let the oppressed go free, and that you break every yoke? (Isaiah 58:6)

In the back section of this journal, I am going to provide some different resources. One of these will be a *Benefits of Fasting* guide. Contrary to belief, it is not a bad thing to be benefit-driven when it comes to certain aspects of our relationship with God. In the end, *He* is our benefit. We pursue Him because of what we get in the exchange: *Him.*

When it comes to fasting, there are tremendous benefits to tapping into this powerful practice, physically *and* spiritually. I want you to be aware of these because it gives you a clear vision of what to expect as you journey on this ten-day transformation.

This is not a workbook where you are going to be answering topical questions. This your opportunity to seek God's face, hear His voice, pray His purposes, and experience His Presence. You get to interact with Him in the pages ahead, as He is the key to our transformation. There is no change apart from Him.

In the next section, you will receive a brief overview of what to expect in the ten days ahead. You will also learn how to use this journal most effectively. We don't want to give you something else to do in an already busy life. I assure you, the minimal time investment you make each day in this journal will yield maximum results in your life.

Whether you go through *Transformation* in community (church, small group), or you are going through it on a more individual level (personal, family), one thing is for sure—the next ten days are going to be an incredible investment into the rest of your life.

Through *Transformation*, I believe God wants to help you:

- Create new, healthy patterns and disciplines in every sphere of your life

- Break addictions, sinful habits, and unhealthy cycles that have held you back from fulfilling your destiny

- Go to a whole new level in your relationship with God

- Experience powerful new dimensions of prayer and Bible study

- See prayers answered and dreams fulfilled that you have nearly given up on

- Step into the next season of His purpose for your life

Get ready to experience some extraordinary things from an extraordinary God!

Many Blessings,

JORDAN RUBIN

INSTRUCTIONS

Instructions on how you may use the Transformation Journal.

NOTE TO LEADERS

If you are leading the *Transformation* experience at your church or with your small group, there will be facilitator instructions available online at www.ChurchAlly.com.

USING THE JOURNAL

There are several different ways you can use this journal.

In a Group Setting

Your small group may end up wanting to go through *Transformation*. It is recommended that your group meets in person at least two times during the ten-day period—preferably three. You should meet on the first day and the last day, but it might be helpful to meet *during* the fast as well for a time of fellowship, encouragement, prayer, and Bible study. Each day between the in-person meetings, you will go through the daily *Transformation* activities on your own.

In a Corporate Church Setting

If your entire church goes through *Transformation*, there is a good chance you will be participating in different daily fast-related activities outside of your *Transformation* journal. Anything your church facilitates is designed to encourage your personal transformation experience and would only add to the benefit you receive going through the journal individually.

DAILY CORPORATE *TRANSFORMATION*

Daily Video Segments

There are several different options for how you can use these brief but encouraging video clips from Jordan:

- You can watch them as a small group before a time of prayer/meeting.

- You can watch them corporately as a church before a time of prayer/meeting.

- You can watch them individually at the beginning of the day or at the end of the day to supplement your reading exercises.

This will be a brief daily prayer directive that your church or small group would be praying about *together*.

We recommend placing these prayer directives on:

- Your church website, so everyone can be praying about the same things at the same times.

- A social networking group that all members of your small group/church could access.

DAILY PERSONAL *TRANSFORMATION*

You will be doing brief exercises in the journal three times a day—morning, afternoon, and evening. The activities should not take you more than five minutes each. You are welcome to go deeper if you have the additional time. These segments are different from the themes explored in the Daily Corporate Transformation sections, as they are intended to help develop a personal routine of Bible study, reflection, and prayer in your life. The topics covered were birthed during one of our original Daniel Fasts, and I believe they are key Truths that will help you spiritually maximize the ten-day transformation. These daily exercises consist of the following:

Scripture

A Scripture verse containing a specific theme for that time of day.

Devotional Thought

A quick devotional thought on how you can apply that Scripture to your everyday life and experience transformation.

Prayer

You get the opportunity to practice the greatest tool of transformation: Prayer. Based on what you read, you now have the opportunity to pray the Word of God over your life and interact with the journal by writing down your prayers, thoughts, and insights.

WHAT IS THE DANIEL DIET?

The Daniel Diet is a partial fast involving the consumption of *only* water and pulse for ten days, seeking God's face in daily prayer three set times per day, and daily Bible study and learning.

The Daniel Diet is based on the first chapter of the Book of Daniel, which describes how Daniel and three young compatriots from Judah were taken into captivity. Instead of consuming the king's delicacies, they asked to consume only foods that the God of Abraham, Isaac, and Jacob had blessed. Paraphrasing from the New King James version, we learn this:

> Please test your servants for ten days, and let them give us pulse to eat and water to drink. Then let our appearance be examined before you.... Then at the end of the ten days, their features appeared better and healthier than all the young men who ate a portion of the king's delicacies.... As for these four youths, God gave them learning and skill in all literature and wisdom.

WHY IS FASTING IMPORTANT?

Now you may be asking *why* it's important to fast.

The answers are numerous, but the main reason to fast, in my opinion, is to receive breakthrough in areas of your life that nothing else can bring and to open doors that cannot be opened by anything else. God reveals this in Isaiah:

Is this not the fast that I have chosen: to loose the bonds of wickedness, to undo the heavy burdens, to let the oppressed go free, and that you break every yoke? ...Then your light shall break forth like the morning, your healing shall spring forth speedily, and your righteousness shall go before you... (Isaiah 58:6,8).

Look at these incredible spiritual benefits of fasting:

1. Fasting can bring you closer to God.

2. Fasting can make you more sensitive to God's voice.

3. Fasting helps break addictions.

4. Fasting shows us our weakness and allows us to rely on God's strength.

Paracelsus, the famed 15th-century physician and alchemist who believed in the body's ability to heal itself, said fasting activates "the Healer within."

Here are some of the incredible emotional benefits of fasting:

1. Fasting helps support healthy emotions.

2. Fasting clears your mind of negative thoughts.

3. Fasting can bring peace.

"There is not a habit or weakness that can survive a siege of prayer and fasting," Edward Earle Purinton wrote in his book, *The Philosophy of Fasting.*

And finally, here are twelve physical benefits of fasting:

1. Fasting helps break addictions to junk food, drinking, and smoking.

2. Fasting supports the body's detoxification systems.

3. Fasting promotes healthy weight loss.

4. Fasting promotes healthy energy levels.

5. Fasting supports healthy aging, healthy skin, and a glowing complexion.

6. Fasting promotes healthy memory, focus, and concentration.

7. Fasting reduces stress and promotes sound sleep.

8. Fasting supports cardiovascular health.

9. Fasting promotes healthy digestion and elimination.

10. Fasting supports healthy inflammation response and promotes joint comfort.

11. Fasting supports healthy immune system function.

12. Fasting promotes healthy hormonal balance.

Dr. Otto H.F. Buchinger, who supervised more than 70,000 fasts, once said, "Fasting is...a royal road to healing for anyone who agrees to take it for the transformation of body, mind, and spirit."

THE BATTLE OF FASTING

Whenever you start a fast, keep this admonition found in Ephesians 6:12 (NIV) in mind: "For our struggle is not against flesh and blood, but against the rulers, against the authorities, against the powers of this dark world and against the spiritual forces of evil in the heavenly realms."

You need to be aware that the enemy knows that if you undertake a fast, then you are about to see an incredible breakthrough in your life, and he wants to stop it. Here are some of the challenges that you may face during your ten-day Daniel Diet:

On the spiritual side:

- Circumstances in your life may seem to be impossible to overcome; this means the fast is working.

- Temptation to break the fast may seem to increase, and you may come up with several "good" reasons to stop it. This means the fast is working.

On the emotional side:

- Because your body will begin throwing off deadly emotions, an initial increase in nervousness, anxiety, and worry may result. This means the fast is working.

On the physical side:

- Since your body will begin to detoxify, you may experience a coated tongue, headaches, bad breath, body odor, digestion and elimination changes, fatigue, and even the sniffles. This means the fast is working.

Two Possible Plans for Your Fast

THE 10-DAY DANIEL DIET

You can follow the Daniel Diet in one of two recommended ways.

OPTION NUMBER 1

Purchase fresh raw fruits, vegetables, nuts, and seeds (organic is preferable) from your local health food or grocery store and consume as outlined below.

You begin by drinking a half-liter of water not long after you wake up. Then be sure to pray at 9 A.M. or at a morning time that's suitable for you.

Your first of three meals is at 12:30 P.M., which consists of one kind of fruit along with healthy fats from avocado, nuts, and seeds and/or coconut. Try to consume only one fruit (two pieces if allowed) and if possible, alternate different fruits each day.

Then some time in the afternoon, approximately 3 P.M., take time to pray, if possible.

At 3:30 P.M., you're going to consume a veggie meal combined with a good source of healthy fats. You can choose any combination of raw veggies. For example, multiple veggies are allowed and should be combined with healthy, high-fat foods such as avocado, coconut (mature, young, or Thai), or raw soaked and sprouted nuts and seeds such as almonds. Fibrous veggies, such as broccoli or cauliflower, can be lightly cooked, although I prefer that you eat your veggies raw if possible.

Can you make a salad? Sure, but since the Daniel Diet nixes the consumption of salt, oils, and sweeteners, this eliminates salad dressings. If you want to make a salad, the way to do it is to toss together greens and add cucumbers, peppers, celery and onions. Then in a blender, throw in avocado, add some chopped onions, raw lemon juice, sliced tomatoes, and hit the power button. What you'll produce is a cross between a dressing, a salad, and a soup. Kind of like a super guacamole, which is delicious on top of your veggies.

At 6:30 P.M., repeat a raw fruit and healthy fat meal with one type of fruit and healthy fats from avocado, coconut, and raw soaked and sprouted nuts and seeds. Throughout the day, make sure to consume between 100 to 128 ounces of pure water per day. This will help facilitate the body's cleansing process. Pray once again in the evening.

Please note that I recommend you skip the traditional breakfast meal and start eating at what would be considered after lunch time each day while following the Daniel Diet.

While you may be used to consuming a large meal shortly upon waking, I believe by narrowing your daily eating time window and thus lengthening your fasting and cleansing time, your health will greatly improve in many ways.

Here is an example of your daily Daniel Diet plan Option Number 1:

- 6:30 A.M.: purified water, 16 ounces

- 8 A.M.: purified water, 16 ounces

- 10 A.M.: purified water, 16 ounces

- 12 P.M.: purified water, 16 ounces

- 12:30 P.M.: grapes (one large bunch), half an avocado, and a handful of raw or soaked almonds and pumpkin seeds

- 2 P.M.: purified water, 16 ounces

- 3:30 P.M.: salad greens, red onion, red peppers, cucumbers, and sprouts topped with a blend of avocado, tomato, red onion, garlic, and lemon juice

- 5 P.M.: purified water, 16 ounces

- 6:30 P.M.: organic fresh strawberries, a half cup of fresh mature coconut or one Thai coconut (you may drink the coconut water), and raw almonds

- 8:00 P.M.: purified water, 16 ounces

You will follow this eating plan on Days 1-9. On Day 10, you should try your best to consume only water and break your Daniel Diet at 5 P.M.

A great way to break the Daniel Diet on the evening of Day 10 is as follows:

- 5 P.M.: drink green vegetable juice (8-16 ounces)

- 5:20 P.M.: consume green salad with organic veggies

- 5:45 P.M.: consume steamed or baked wild fish such as salmon

- 8 P.M.: drink a smoothie

SMOOTHIE RECIPE

8 oz. plain Amasai, yogurt (goat or sheep milk), or kefir (goat or sheep milk)	1 tablespoon extra-virgin coconut oil
2 raw eggs (organic pasture-raised), optional	1 tablespoon raw almond butter (optional)
1 fresh banana	1 tablespoon cacao powder (optional)
½ avocado	3 tablespoons Terrain Omega or milled sprouted seeds
1 tablespoon raw unheated honey	
vanilla extract, to taste (alcohol extract, not glycerin)	

OPTION NUMBER 2

There's another way you can follow the ten-day Daniel Diet that's super convenient, healthy, and delicious. Beyond Organic has created EA Pulse, which are enzyme-activated organic superfood meals that will power your Daniel Diet. These include raw, sprouted organic fruits, vegetables, nuts, and seeds, and fermented living herbs.

Loaded with antioxidants, fiber, vitamins, minerals, omega-3 fats, probiotics, and enzymes from over thirty superfoods, each EA Pulse blend may be one of the most nutrient-dense meals you've ever consumed. We combine EA Pulse with Terrain Tonic 10, a botanically infused structured water containing ten treasured botanicals that were widely consumed in the days of Daniel and considered as or more valuable than precious metals.

For about the same price the average American spends on food per day, you can have all of your Daniel Diet foods and beverages shipped directly to your door. For more information on the Daniel Diet 10-Day Transformation Pack, visit www.LiveBeyondOrganic.com.

Here is an example of your daily Daniel Diet plan that is Option Number 2:

- 6:30 A.M.: drink one bottle (16 ounces) of Terrain Tonic 10 (botanically infused structured water)

- 8 A.M.: drink one bottle (16 ounces) of Terrain Tonic 10 (botanically infused structured water)

- 10 A.M.: drink one bottle (16 ounces) of Terrain Tonic 10 (botanically infused structured water)

- 12:30 P.M.: one bag of EA Pulse Antioxidant Fruits (see ingredient list below)

- 2 P.M.: drink one bottle (16 ounces) of Terrain Tonic 10 (botanically infused structured water)

- 3:30 P.M.: consume one bag of EA Pulse Super Veggies (see ingredient list below)

- 4:30 P.M.: drink one bottle (16 ounces) of Terrain Tonic 10 (botanically infused structured water)

- 6 P.M.: drink one bottle (16 ounces) of Terrain Tonic 10 (botanically infused structured water)

- 6:30 P.M.: consume one bag of EA Pulse Omega Fruits (see ingredient list below)

- 8:00 P.M.: drink one bottle (16 ounces) of Terrain Tonic 10 (botanically infused structured water)

You will follow this eating plan on Days 1-9. On Day 10, you should try your best to consume six bottles Terrain Tonic 10 and break your Daniel Diet partial fast at 5 P.M.

A great way to break the Daniel Diet on the evening of Day 10 is as follows. Note that many of the foods and beverages listed below are available at www.LiveBeyondOrganic.com.

- 5 P.M.: drink 8-16 ounces of SueroViv (green is best)

- 5:20 P.M.: consume a green salad with organic veggies, Beyond Organic Greenfed Cheese, and EA Live Seven Seed Crackers

- 5:45 P.M.: consume a Beyond Organic Green-Finished Ranch Roast, sautéed veggies with sweet potato or quinoa

- 8 P.M.: drink an EA Live Smoothie (which will be like a thick pudding)

EA LIVE SMOOTHIE RECIPE

8 oz. plain Amasai	1 tablespoon raw, unheated honey
2 raw eggs (organic pasturer	vanilla extract to taste (alcohol
1 fresh banana	extract, not glycerin)
½ avocado	1 tablespoon extra-virgin coconut oil
3 tablespoons (1 serving) Terrain Omega	1 tablespoon raw almond butter (optional)
or EA Live Sprouted Seven Blend	1 tablespoon raw cacao powder (optional)

Or you can consume EA Live Granola with Amasai (plain). (See Appendix D for EA Pulse Ingredient Listing).

FLEX OPTIONS FOR THE DANIEL DIET

The Daniel Diet may be the most effective cleanse available, but it can also be extremely challenging. If you find yourself having a difficult time sticking to the program but really want to persevere, we offer the follow flex options.

During the ten-day Daniel Diet, if your appetite and/or food cravings are getting the best of you, or if you find yourself experiencing unbearable detoxification symptoms such as loose bowels, aches, pains, fatigue, etc., we offer five flex meals.

While I believe the best results are achieved by following one of the two Daniel Diet options listed above, you may consume five flex meals during your ten-day Daniel Diet. The Flex Meal should occur in place of your third meal of the day, starting at 6:30 P.M. and ending at 7:30 P.M. It's important to consume the meal within the one-hour allotted time period. Each flex meal can consist of foods from one of three categories with Number 1 being optimal and Number 2 and Number 3 being acceptable alternatives:

1.   Consume any raw, fresh organic fruit, vegetable, nut, seed, or raw/cold-pressed vegetable oil (i.e. extra-virgin olive oil)

2.   Consume any combination of raw or cooked vegetable, fruit, nut, seed, or gluten-free whole grain (soaked and

sprouted is best). Examples are amaranth, quinoa, millet, and buckwheat. You may also consume high mineral sea salt.

3.   Consume any biblically correct food from the correct food from the food list in *The Maker's Diet Revolution*, pages 213-225.

Our goal for you during this 10-Day Daniel Diet is to experience wonderful results while feeling your best. While some will have no trouble following one of the two Daniel Diet protocols exactly as written, our goal is for everyone to have a successful and comfortable experience while cleansing. Since the concept of fasting is so foreign to our modern culture and diet, the flex meals ensure virtually anyone can follow the Daniel Diet to completion.

SOME FINAL FASTING INSTRUCTIONS

Please note that I encourage you to refrain from any other foods, beverages, or other commonly consumed items during this ten-day period. This includes but is not limited to coffee, energy drinks, gum, mints, or candy.

If you are on medication and/or under the care of a physician, please consult him or her before beginning this or any diet regimen, *and by no means* should you alter your medication dosage or schedule. Please check the ingredients for each of the EA Pulse products, and do not undertake the 10-Day Daniel Diet if you have known allergies to any of the ingredients.

THE DANIEL DIET DARE

Goals: As a Daniel Diet participant, you're encouraged to set goals (via a 500-word essay) that you'd like to see God accomplish in and through your life in the areas of physical, spiritual, mental, and emotional health.

The Diet: You will be undertaking the Daniel Diet inspired by Daniel 1:12. I was inspired to develop this ten-day diet that I believe accurately represents the diet that Daniel, Hananiah (Shadrach), Misha-el (Meshach), and Azariah (Abednego) consumed—in order to honor God—while they were held in Babylonian captivity.

Prayer: Commit to daily prayer three times per day—both corporately and individually.

Results: You can expect to see fantastic transformation in body, mind, and spirit as God gives you ten times the wisdom, favor, and understanding as husbands, wives, mothers, and fathers, as well as in your leadership, business, job, school, service, athletics, and all areas of your life.

There's another idea I want to share, and I file this under the category of "extra credit." I want to encourage you to "fast" from the popular culture and take a respite from watching TV, surfing for hours on the Internet, and all the "noise" that threatens to sabotage our lives.

You might look at the Daniel Diet as a time to study or practice something you've always wanted to learn. Maybe there's a book on an important topic (such as child-rearing) that you've always wanted to read but never seem to have time for. Perhaps this is your chance to finally listen to those Spanish DVDs from Rosetta Stone that you purchased at the airport but never got around to using. Or maybe this is your time to learn to play a musical instrument.

I hope by now you can see that there are so many compelling reasons to take ten days out of your busy schedule to transform your body, mind, and spirit by following the Daniel Diet.

Day One

REPENTANCE

CORPORATE PRAYER TRANSFORMATION

If we confess our sins, He is faithful and just to forgive us our sins and to cleanse us from all unrighteousness (1 John 1:9).

There are two sides of repentance and one cannot exist without the other. First, we must closely examine our lives and ask the Lord to reveal any sin that we have been holding onto. Remember, God does not want to condemn you; He came to cleanse you! Jesus paid a high price so that you could follow I John 1:9 and receive the power of its promise in your life today. First, confess your sins before the Father without fear of condemnation. Second, the Scripture assures us that as we do this, God is "faithful and just to forgive us our sins and cleanse us from all unrighteousness." We experience confidence that we are cleansed and righteous when we are bold enough to confess our sins before an ever-loving, always-forgiving Father.

- Repent without condemnation! Instead, repent of sin and incorrect thinking, knowing that the Holy Spirit wants to produce in you the very mind of Christ, so that in every situation you are able to deal with it as Jesus would.

- Repent for the sin in your life and ask the Lord to become more satisfying and pleasurable to you than sin.

- Repent for not thinking like God does, and in turn, ask for the Holy Spirit to form within you the very mind of Christ.

- Repent for not thinking that God is actually as good as His Word reveals Him to be—His goodness leads to repentance.

- Confess anything in your life that might be displeasing to God, and receive the forgiveness Jesus purchased with His blood on the cross.

- Repent for the areas where you are not pursuing God's best for your life, and ask the Holy Spirit to give you fresh vision on your purpose and destiny.

Day One

DELIVERER

Daily Personal Transformation

Morning | The Lord Who Delivered...*Will Deliver*

Scripture

> *Moreover David said, "The Lord, who delivered me from the paw of the lion and from the paw of the bear, He will deliver me from the hand of this Philistine"* (1 Samuel 17:37).

Devotional

When David stood before the giant, Goliath, he approached the taunting Philistine with great confidence because he knew that the God who delivered him in the past—from the lion and from the bear—would deliver him again. Never underestimate the power of testimony in positioning you to stand victoriously against future trials and impossibilities. Whatever you are facing now, come against it with confidence and strength, reminding yourself of God's track record of victory in your life.

Prayer Journal

What are some "giants" facing your life today? List your current "giants," and beside them, list times in your life (or even in Scripture) where God brought victory to similar situations. Remember, if He *delivered*, He *will deliver*!

_____

_____

_____

_____

_____

_____

_____

AFTERNOON | TRUST THE LORD AND RELY ON HIS WISDOM

Scripture

Do not be wise in your own eyes; fear the Lord and shun evil. This will bring health to your body and nourishment to your bones (Proverbs 3:7-8 NIV).

Devotional

All of us want to be in control. It is especially easy to want control when we are dealing with situations in our lives that seem to be going out of control. The reality is, there is only One who possesses true wisdom on how to best handle these situations, and that is the Lord. When we are wise in our own eyes, we are basically telling God, "I know how to handle this best." That could not be farther from the truth. Imagine if David used natural, human wisdom coming against Goliath? It would have been disastrous. He surrendered his natural, human wisdom to God's and experienced history-making victory.

Give God control today over every area of your life. Remember, He is completely trustworthy and desires nothing but good for you. The Lord who *delivered* will faithfully deliver again!

Prayer Journal

What are some areas in your life that you need to surrender to God that you have been trying to fix in your own strength or wisdom? (Ask the Lord to reveal these to you and list them out. You will return to this list this evening.)

_____

_____

_____

_____

_____

_____

_____

EVENING | EXPERIENCING THE BEYOND-COMPREHENSION PEACE OF GOD

Scripture

Be anxious for nothing, but in everything by prayer and supplication with thanksgiving let your requests be made known to God. And the peace of God, which surpasses all comprehension, will guard your hearts and your minds in Christ Jesus (Philippians 4:6-7 NASB).

Devotional

Remember the list you made this afternoon—specifically, the items you need to turn over to God? He does not want you to be anxious about any of those things. In fact, He wants you to live in a state of dialogue (prayer) with Him about those things that have the tendency to make people anxious, worried, and fearful. As you get ready to sleep tonight, remember that instead of anxiety and fear, the will of God is for you to walk in peace that surpasses all comprehension.

How do you walk in this supernatural peace? Trust Him with every situation in your life. Every anxiety. Every fear. Every impossibility facing you this evening. Cast all of these things upon the Lord, for He truly, deeply cares for you! (See I Peter 5:7.)

Prayer Journal

Go back to the list you made this afternoon.

Bring each of these items to God in prayer, releasing them to Him. Remember, once you give them to God, they are His. Don't try to take them back.

They are no longer on your "to do" list; they are now on God's.

After you release your cares and concerns to God in prayer, begin thanking Him for how He is already moving in each situation.

Thank Him for the supernatural peace that He is filling your heart and mind with—even at this very moment!

Day Two

SPIRITUAL AWAKENING

CORPORATE PRAYER DIRECTIVE

Therefore He says: "Awake, you who sleep, arise from the dead, and Christ will give you light" (Ephesians 5:14).

As our hearts are now in a position of repentance, with minds that desire to be transformed by the Holy Spirit, we are in a place of awakening. More than God sending something down from heaven (another revival or outpouring of the Holy Spirit), His agenda for these last days involves us, His church, living awakened *lifestyles*. God is making it more and more clear that revival is not an event; it is a transformed lifestyle.

The things that tend to characterize revival were never meant to be limited to a single event or timeframe. This is the normal Christian life. What is God's will for our lives? Simple—model Jesus Christ in His love, compassion, and power.

- Pray for personal awakening, that your passion would be fixed on Jesus.

- Pray for personal renewal, that the Holy Spirit would remind you of God's specific purpose for your life and His grand purpose—to model Jesus Christ.

- Pray that God would settle in your heart the truth that revival is not an experience or event; you carry revival because you carry His presence!

- Pray that God would embolden your spirit, reminding you that you carry His Kingdom, you are His house, and you are indwelt by His presence.

Day Two

PROVIDER AND PROTECTOR

DAILY PERSONAL TRANSFORMATION

MORNING | FORGET NOT HIS BENEFITS!

Scripture

> *Praise the Lord, my soul; all my inmost being, praise his holy name. Praise the Lord, my soul, and forget not all his benefits— who forgives all your sins and heals all your diseases, who redeems your life from the pit and crowns you with love and compassion, who satisfies your desires with good things so that your youth is renewed like the eagle's* (Psalms 103:1-5 NIV).

Devotional

We are actually instructed *not* to forget all of the benefits that come as a result of a relationship with the Lord. It's almost like David is giving us a command here! We do a great job emphasizing the fact that we do not serve God just because of what we get out of it, but we serve Him because He is worthy—and the Cross was enough.

This is absolutely true. At the same time, to actually live a victorious Christian life, we need to learn how to access every single benefit God has made available to us. Refuse to live below the benefits that the Lord has provided you. Access them. Enjoy them. Watch them release the supernatural in your life—during this ten-day experience and beyond!

Prayer Journal

Based on the benefits listed in Psalm 103:1-5, which ones do you need to access and experience in your life *today?* Write them down, and thank the Lord for making them available to you and for releasing them in your life.

_____

_____

_____

_____

_____

_____

AFTERNOON | DWELLING IN THE MOST HIGH

Scripture

He who dwells in the secret place of the Most High shall abide under the shadow of the Almighty. I will say of the Lord, "He is my refuge and my fortress; my God, in Him I will trust" (Psalms 91:1-2).

Devotional

Psalm 91 reminds us that God's desire is to supernaturally protect His people. The key is, we need to make the Lord, the *Most High*, our dwelling place. In the midst of confusion, catastrophe, and difficult situations, it is amazing how we are quick to dwell on a variety of different things—most of which are unproductive and unfruitful. Fear and worry involve us dwelling on all of those possible negative outcomes. God does not want us dwelling on fear, but rather, dwelling in faith in Him.

How do we do this? We focus on His promises—what His Word says. Regardless of what is coming against you today, remember, your dwelling place is the *Most High* and His promises are higher than any situation that might be coming against your life. He is your Rock and Strong Tower from the enemy (see Ps. 61:3).

Prayer Journal

At the end of our daily directives, we have included the entire chapter of Psalm 91. Review it throughout the day, as you are able. Identify specific promises that you need to focus on. Trade any fear you might be experiencing for faith in the truth of God's Word (see Psalm 91).

_____

_____

_____

_____

_____

_____

_____

EVENING | FILLED TO THE FULL

Scripture

> *And my God will liberally supply* (fill to the full) *your every need according to His riches in glory in Christ Jesus* (Philippians 4:19 AMP).

Devotional

This recent season in history has been a time of great instability for the nations of the earth. At the same time, we do not live our lives based on what is going on in the world around us, as we are citizens of heaven. We are ambassadors, called to represent Christ in this world.

As a result, we offer hope to an on-looking world. We give the world the picture of a people who are taken care of and are abundantly provided for, even when everything looks bleak, hopeless, and spiraling downward. This speaks loudly of God's faithfulness. Remember, God wants to provide for all of your needs; yes, for your sake and personal benefit, but also as a testimony of His goodness to a world that so desperately needs to know Him. Let's never forget that our personal blessing is a testimony that reveals who He is and what He is like to the nations (see Ps. 67:1-2).

Prayer Journal

What are some specific needs you have (physical, financial, relational, emotional, etc.) that you need the Lord to provide for? How can His blessing in these areas be a testimony to the people who are watching your life and walk with the Lord?

_____

_____

_____

_____

_____

_____

He who dwells in the secret place of the Most High Shall abide under the shadow of the Almighty. I will say of the Lord, "He is my refuge and my fortress; My God, in Him I will trust."

Surely He shall deliver you from the snare of the fowler And from the perilous pestilence. He shall cover you with His feathers, And under His wings you shall take refuge; His truth shall be your shield and buckler. You shall not be afraid of the terror by night, Nor of the arrow that flies by day, Nor of the pestilence that walks in darkness, Nor of the destruction that lays waste at noonday.

A thousand may fall at your side, And ten thousand at your right hand; But it shall not come near you. Only with your eyes shall you look, And see the reward of the wicked.

Because you have made the Lord, who is my refuge, Even the Most High, your dwelling place, No evil shall befall you, Nor shall any plague come near your dwelling; For He shall give His angels charge over you, To keep you in all your ways. In their hands they shall bear you up, Lest you dash your foot against a stone. You shall tread upon the lion and the cobra, The young lion and the serpent you shall trample underfoot.

"Because he has set his love upon Me, therefore I will deliver him; I will set him on high, because he has known My name. He shall call upon Me, and I will answer him; I will be with him in trouble; I will deliver him and honor him. With long life I will satisfy him, And show him My salvation" (Psalms 91:1-16).

Day Three

FOCUS ON JESUS

CORPORATE PRAYER DIRECTIVE

Therefore we also, since we are surrounded by so great a cloud of witnesses, let us lay aside every weight, and the sin which so easily ensnares us, and let us run with endurance the race that is set before us, looking unto Jesus, the author and finisher of our faith... (Hebrews 12:1-2).

Once we repent from our sins and recognize the need to live an awakened lifestyle, the question is: *How do we live a transformed lifestyle? What is our model? What is God's will?* It is all wrapped up in the Person of Jesus Christ. We need to be the rare people in this generation who continue to keep our eyes fixed on Jesus, not looking to the left or the right. There are so many distractions in life—so many voices competing for our attention. In this time of corporate fasting and prayer, let us be committed to beholding Jesus like never before, for He is truly the example of the normal Christian life.

- Pray for continued focus on Jesus as the central part of our lives, our families, and our future.

- Pray that as our focus on Him increases that our clarity in other areas of life would also increase.

- Pray that Jesus would be the focus of our families.

- Pray that Jesus would be the focus of our careers, jobs, and business.

- Pray that we would not be distracted by the messages and voices of the world and simply look to Jesus as the model for how to live.

- Pray that Jesus would be displayed in compassion, love, and power through your awakened, transformed life.

Day Three

HIS STRENGTH, YOUR VICTORY

DAILY PERSONAL TRANSFORMATION

MORNING | *THROUGH* THE VALLEY

Scripture

> *Yea, though I walk through the valley of the shadow of death, I will fear no evil: for thou art with me...* (Psalms 23:4 KJV).

Devotional

So many of us are familiar with Psalm 23 as a timeless word of comfort. I also want to share with you a powerful word of encouragement that this treasured Psalm offers, not just for the life to come, but for the here and now. Notice that David writes, *I walk through the valley*. He did not make plans to give up, lie down, and die in the valley; he was intent on going through. How? His strength was in the Good Shepherd who walked beside Him. The same Shepherd who walked with David through many, many dark valleys is with you today. Be encouraged, for the Shepherd of David is your Strength and He will walk *through* the valley with you and bring you to the other side.

Prayer Journal

What valleys do you feel like you are going through today? Specifically: Are there certain situations in your life that you feel like you have been walking in for a long time, with no end in sight?

Write these down and commit to praying for breakthrough in this time of prayer and fasting. Remember, fasting has the ability to release breakthrough and open doors that normal methods do not.

_____

_____

_____

_____

_____

_____

_____

AFTERNOON | YOUR TRIALS, HIS TESTIMONIES

Scripture

Consider it pure joy, my brothers and sisters, whenever you face trials of many kinds, because you know that the testing of your faith produces perseverance. Let perseverance finish its work so that you may be mature and complete, not lacking anything (James 1:2-4 NIV).

Devotional

We need to change the way we view *trials of many kinds*. They are unpleasant, I know. They consume our energy, our thought lives, and our emotions. Trials are an unavoidable part of the human experience. That said, I do believe we can change our perspective when it comes to how we observe trials in our lives. This is what James is encouraging us to do. How in the world can we observe trials as a joy?

We cannot treat the trial as our conqueror. Remember, on the other side of the valley is victory. We go *through*. Your trials are setups for your testimonies, and those testimonies of victory, breakthrough, and answered prayer are not purposed only bless our lives, but as we share testimonies, they encourage others to believe that if God got us through our trials, He can do the same for them.

Prayer Journal

What are some trials you need to change your perspective on?

As God answers these prayers for *you*, bringing breakthrough and victory, how will your testimony encourage other people in your life who need to experience God in the same way?

_____

_____

_____

_____

_____

_____

_____

EVENING | ANCHORS OF PROMISE

Scripture

"He himself bore our sins" in his body on the cross, so that we might die to sins and live for righteousness; "by his wounds you have been healed" (1 Peter 2:24 NIV).

Devotional

Trials are inevitable, and yes, we have a positive expectation that a testimony will come out of the trial. But the question remains: How do I make it *through*? You might be thinking: *I'm in the trial right now. What do I do in the meantime?* We go *through* the valley. We go *through* the trials. *Through* is what we need to figure out. In my own life, God got me through the valley of disease by giving me an anchor of promise. For me, I Peter 2:24 was that anchor, which reminded me that no matter what I was going through or how bad I felt, Jesus had purchased my healing. Through my valley, this verse of promise was my strength. I want to encourage you to find anchors of promise in Scripture that help you hold fast while going *through* your valley on your way to victory.

Prayer Journal

Take some time to find promises in Scripture that give you an "anchor" for the trials you are currently going through.

Ask the Holy Spirit to guide you through the Word and help you find these verses. Write them down and make them your personal anchors of promise as you continue through the trials.

_____

_____

_____

_____

_____

_____

Day Four

LIVE THE TRUTH

CORPORATE PRAYER DIRECTIVE

Therefore, I urge you, brothers and sisters, in view of God's mercy, to offer your bodies as a living sacrifice, holy and pleasing to God—THIS IS YOUR TRUE AND PROPER WORSHIP. Do not conform to the pattern of this world, but be transformed by the renewing of your mind. Then you will be able to test and approve what God's will is—his good, pleasing and perfect will (Romans 12:1-2 NIV).

Following Jesus' example is more demanding than wearing a bracelet or having a bumper sticker on the back of your car. It is possible to have some of the externals of Christianity, but yet live a lifestyle that is still the same as everyone else who does not know Christ. To live a transformed lifestyle, we need to live "in view of God's mercy" through Jesus. We are motivated to follow Jesus with complete abandon and total obedience when we live in constant view of the mercy God provided for us at the Cross. In response to His work, we offer our lives as living sacrifices. How could we not after what He did for us? He gave everything, and when we constantly remind ourselves of this, it becomes quite natural for us to willingly give everything for Him. Remember, it is one thing to know, and even confess a truth; it's an entirely different thing to live it out. Let's take our place as a trans-formed people and live out the Truth in our everyday lives.

- Pray you will be reminded of the redemptive work of Jesus—constantly living "in view" of His mercy.

- Pray for boldness to stand for the Truth, even when it is not popular and it becomes difficult.

- Pray for grace and strength—that you would refuse to compromise on the standards in God's Word, even when it seems like everyone else is.

- Pray for the Truth of God's Word to be lived out in your everyday life, not just in talk, but in deed and action.

- Pray that your lifestyle testifies to the Truth and points others toward a relationship with Jesus.

Day Four

WISDOM

DAILY PERSONAL TRANSFORMATION

MORNING | WISDOM...WITH EXPECTATION

Scripture

> *If any of you lacks wisdom, let him ask of God, who gives to all liberally and without reproach, and it will be given to him. But let him ask in faith, with no doubting, for he who doubts is like a wave of the sea driven and tossed by the wind* (James 1:5-6).

Devotional

All of us need wisdom. From making daily decisions to navigating some of the more difficult seasons of life, wisdom is a certain common denominator. We need to be sure that when we approach God, asking for wisdom, we don't simply offer up a prayer or cry for help, but rather, we ask with *expectation*.

In fact, James tells us that the key to accessing and receiving wisdom from God is to ask *in faith*. Too often, we throw up prayers to God out of habit, but there is no expectation of an answer attached to the prayer. When it comes to wisdom, let's start being intentional. You *can* pray for wisdom and actually expect to receive it!

Prayer Journal

What are some specific decisions or situations you need wisdom for? Write these down and pray with expectation, believing that God *will* give you wisdom for each one.

As the wisdom comes for these situations, write down what the Holy Spirit shares with you concerning each item on your list.

Perhaps it comes in a way you did not expect, but you sense God is in it. Perhaps it defies logic or natural thought, but you sense the peace of God in the answer you are receiving and it is in agreement with God's Word. Write it all down, pray about it, and begin to put it to work!

_____

_____

_____

_____

_____

_____

_____

AFTERNOON | WISDOM TO KNOW
AND DO GOD'S WILL

Scripture

Rejoice always, pray without ceasing, in everything give thanks; for this is the will of God in Christ Jesus for you (1 Thessalonians 5:16-18).

Devotional

One of the most popular questions asked by believers and non-believers alike is this: *What is my purpose?* In Christian circles, we phrase it this way: "What is God's will for my life?" I believe that the apostle Paul gives us some wisdom concerning this matter. He writes that God's will is for us to rejoice always, pray without ceasing, and continually give thanks. Doing these three things actually opens a door for the Lord to release specific wisdom and direction into our lives and give us greater understanding of the unique calling He has assigned for us. The problem is many of us are seeking the specific without even doing the general! Let's start here, and move forward with expectation that God will release wisdom concerning His plans and purposes for our lives.

Prayer Journal

Pray about the following three things and ask the Holy Spirit to give you vision for what each of these looks like in your life. As you receive inspiration, write down your thoughts:

What does it look like to *rejoice always?*

_____

_____

_____

_____

How can you *pray without ceasing?*

_____

_____

_____

_____

In what ways can you *give thanks* in every situation?

_____

_____

_____

_____

EVENING | WISDOM TO PERSEVERE

Scripture

> *Anyone who meets a testing challenge head-on and manages to stick it out is mighty fortunate. For such persons loyally in love with God, the reward is life and more life* (James 1:12 MSG).

Devotional

As we have been studying wisdom, one of the most important areas in life that we need to pray for and expect God's wisdom is in perseverance. We need to know how to keep moving forward, trusting and believing God, even when everything around us seems dark and does not make any sense. This is where we deal with two types of wisdom—worldly wisdom and godly wisdom. Worldly wisdom gives up, for it observes trials as insurmountable. Worldly wisdom is actually what labels things as impossible and hopeless.

The wisdom of God, on the other hand, gives you everything you need to face challenges *head-on*. God's wisdom gives you *His* perspective. His wisdom gives you specific Scripture anchors to cling on to. His wisdom gives you hope when everything feels hopeless. His wisdom reminds you that on the other side of the trial is *life and more life*. To see from this perspective and persevere, you need God's wisdom. How wonderful to know that God's wisdom is only a prayer away?

Prayer Journal

Take this opportunity to pray for other people in your life who are going through trials. Pray specifically that they experience the wisdom of God to persevere and get to the other side.

Write down their names here and continue to pray for their situations until they experience breakthrough:

_____

_____

_____

_____

_____

_____

_____

Day Five

HEALING AND WHOLENESS

CORPORATE PRAYER DIRECTIVE

Who Himself bore our sins in His own body on the tree, that we, having died to sins, might live for righteousness—BY WHOSE STRIPES YOU WERE HEALED (1 Peter 2:24).

Wholeness is God's perfect will for humanity. I stand as living proof of this. If you need any kind of healing in your life, whether it would be physical, emotional, or spiritual, God the Father has made provision for you to experience completeness because of Jesus. This is the *Shalom* of God. More than just a nice greeting or statement of "peace," Shalom speaks of God's wholeness flowing to every area of our lives. We live in a broken world. Sin is responsible for this sad state, and ultimately, complete and full healing will come when Jesus Himself sets up His reign on the earth. Until then, however, we are called to press in to experience God's healing power in the here and now. Whether you personally need healing, or there are friends and family members you think of who need God's touch, let's get ready to experience the Shalom of heaven in every area of our lives.

- Pray that you and your family walk in divine health—spirit, soul, and body.

- Pray that you would be disciplined to make consistent good choices in food, exercise, and overall lifestyle decisions.

- Pray for divine healing for those who are facing an attack of sickness from the enemy.

- Pray for miracles and healings to occur in the lives of those who don't know Jesus as a sign that points them to receive the good news of the Gospel.

- Pray that God would use you as an instrument of His healing power.

- Pray for discernment as you go through your daily life, asking the Holy Spirit to lead you into divine connections where you have opportunities to release God's power into impossible and broken situations.

Day Five

LISTEN

DAILY PERSONAL TRANSFORMATION

MORNING | BE QUICK TO LISTEN

Scripture

Understand this, my dear brothers and sisters: You must all be quick to listen, slow to speak, and slow to get angry (James 1:19 NLT).

Devotional

I'm not sure why it has become so easy to do the opposite of what this verse talks about. However, we must learn to listen before we speak. This is invaluable when it comes to creating healthy relationships on earth, but also, this principle significantly impacts how we relate with our heavenly Father. Prayer has become identified by what we say. Quite frankly, it should be the opposite. May we be quick to listen to His voice before we start speaking.

Think about it. How much more effective would our prayers be if they were *informed* by what God was saying? Do you want to pray with greater power and effectiveness, seeing more results? Apply James 1:19. In the place of prayer, listen to His voice first, and then pray what you hear Him saying. I promise, as you listen to God's voice and pray what He is saying, you will hit the mark *every time!*

Prayer Journal

Before you start praying today, spend a few moments in God's Presence first, listening for His voice. Ask Him how He would like you to pray. Ask the Holy Spirit if there are things He wants you to pray for. Ask Him how to pray.

Write down what you believe the Lord wants you to be praying for:

_____

_____

_____

_____

_____

_____

_____

AFTERNOON | GETTING QUIET AND LISTENING TO GOD'S HEARTBEAT

Scripture

If anyone among you thinks he is religious, and does not bridle his tongue but deceives his own heart, this one's religion is useless. Pure and undefiled religion before God and the Father is this: to visit orphans and widows in their trouble, and to keep oneself unspotted from the world (James 1:26-27).

Devotional

Our priorities are defined in the place of quiet listening to the Lord's voice. It is so easy when we are constantly talking and doing and working to get off track. There is balance. Yes, we need to talk. We need to declare the Good News. We need to do what the Lord has given us to do. The problem comes when there is no balance between listening and doing. When we move into a lifestyle of all talk, our Christianity can start to become "all talk" and no substance. When we slow down and listen, we begin to hear God's heartbeat and it's in those intimate moments of listening that we hear what is most important to God. This includes, but is not limited to: visiting orphans, taking care of widows, and keeping ourselves clean from the world's contamination.

Prayer Journal

Spend this time in prayer *listening, not talking.*

Ask the Lord for what is on His heart and listen with open ears. He might reveal something right then and there; He may do so later. Be sure to remain in this attitude all day, as the Holy Spirit wants it to become a way you consistently approach God in prayer.

_____

_____

_____

_____

_____

_____

_____

EVENING | HEARING AND RELEASING HEAVEN

Scripture

> *Your kingdom come. Your will be done on earth as it is in heaven* (Matthew 6:10).

Devotional

Before Jesus introduces the Lord's Prayer, He talks about how we should approach the place of prayer. He was not presenting some legalistic protocol, but rather, giving us a perspective. In the prayer discussion, Jesus describes a *secret place* (see Matt. 6:6). I believe this is the quiet place where we hear God's voice, access His heart, and receive His vision.

Jesus modeled a lifestyle of listening to the Father. He was 100 percent God, but He also lived as a man, and throughout His ministry, He constantly talked about how He only said what He heard the Father saying. May we do the same. The result? We will see God's will done, *on earth*, as we pray the things that are in line His will and His heart.

Prayer Journal

Ask the Holy Spirit to give you vision for the things God wants to release into the earth *through you*.

Day Six

LIFE AND DEATH

CORPORATE PRAYER DIRECTIVE

Death and life are in the power of the tongue... (Proverbs 18:21).

We need to learn how to speak God's truth, not the world's lies. Too many of us spend a lot of our time agreeing with the world with our words. We may think we are doing our best to live a Christ-following lifestyle, but in the end, one of the greatest factors that betrays a lifestyle of true discipleship is how we speak. Do the words that come out of our mouths agree with culture and the lies of the enemy that define the world, or do they agree with the Word of God—even if everything in our lives and everything around us appears contrary to the very Scripture we are saying? Let's be known as a people who speak life, not death. We speak hope, not discouragement. This is not fanciful, "think happy thoughts, speak positive words" theology. This is a call to really line up every area of our lives with the Word of God, and one of the key areas to do this is through our speech.

- Pray that your words would build people up, not tear them down.

- Pray that when people hear you speak, your words minister life to them.

- Pray that your words would release healing, hope, and encouragement.

- Pray that you would think before you speak, making sure that your words are a good representation of Jesus.

- Pray that you would be mindful not to speak like the world, but instead, like an ambassador of God's Kingdom.

Day Six

FAITH AND ACTION

DAILY PERSONAL TRANSFORMATION

MORNING | TAKING STEPS TO DEMONSTRATE FAITH

Scripture

> In the same way, faith by itself, if it is not accompanied by action, is dead (James 2:17 NIV).

Devotional

By faith Abraham left his homeland to go out to the place he would receive as an inheritance, not knowing where he was going (see Heb. 11:8). By faith Abraham offered up Isaac (see Heb. 11:17-19). Because of Abraham's actions that accompanied his faith, God knew what was in Abraham's heart (fear and love for God).

After Abraham took steps of faith, God came through and provided land for Abraham and a ram for him to sacrifice instead of Isaac. One of God's names is Jehovah Jireh, which means "The Lord Will Provide" (see Gen. 22:14). Sometimes we have to take steps of faith in order to see the Lord provide for us.

Prayer Journal

What are steps of faith you feel the Lord is asking you to take?

——————————————————————————

——————————————————————————

——————————————————————————

——————————————————————————

——————————————————————————

——————————————————————————

AFTERNOON | DON'T CONFORM, BE TRANSFORMED

Scripture

> Do not conform to the pattern of this world, but be transformed
> by the renewing of your mind. Then you will be able to test and
> approve what God's will is—his good, pleasing and perfect will
> (Romans 12:1-2 NIV).

Devotional

When we align our beliefs and actions with Kingdom principles, we most likely won't look like the world looks. We will be conformed and transformed into the image of Christ! A byproduct of this is that people will see Jesus in us by the way we act.

The world is searching for truth, and you might be the only Jesus somebody meets. Let your life be a living sacrifice to God, knowing that you will be simultaneously witnessing to the world around you.

Prayer Journal

Are there some areas of your life you sense God wants to transform? It could be renewing your mind and changing the way you think, or it could be changing the way you interact with someone, or it could even be changing the way you spend money. Take a moment to ask God what He wants you to change in your life as a sacrifice to Him.

_____

_____

_____

_____

_____

_____

_____

EVENING | SUBMIT TO GOD AND RESIST TEMPTATION

Scripture

Therefore submit to God. Resist the devil and he will flee from you. Draw near to God and He will draw near to you... (James 4:7-8).

Devotional

Temptation can seem overwhelming at times, but remember that you don't have to struggle against the devil or temptation on your own. With God you are *more than a conqueror*! There is no comparison between God's power and the enemy's power to tempt you. God is infinitely more powerful! Because you are God's child, His power is available for you to draw from. The key is to "submit to God" and "draw near to God" by asking Him for help.

Prayer Journal

Are there some areas you are struggling with temptation? Acknowledge that God is able to help you and ask Him for help each time that temptation arises. He will give you creative strategies to overcome. You can ask Him ahead of time for a plan of action. Maybe it is declaring Scripture out loud, or maybe it is worshiping the Lord, or maybe it is praying for an unsaved friend.

Submit yourself to God through prayer now by acknowledging that He is all-powerful, and then ask Him to help you overcome temptation. Ask Him for a creative strategy to resist temptation and write it down.

_____

_____

_____

_____

_____

_____

Day Seven

GOD'S PROTECTION

CORPORATE PRAYER DIRECTIVE

He shall cover you with His feathers, and under His wings you shall take refuge; His truth shall be your shield and buckler (Psalms 91:4).

One of the keys to walking in God's protection is found in verse 4, where we see that *His truth shall be your shield and buckler*. In the midst of life's circumstances and storms, our assurance of protection comes from knowing and resting in God's Word—His eternal and unchanging Truth. The New Living Translation puts it this way: "His faithful promises are your armor and protection." When we become consumed with the trials of life but are not focused on the promises contained in God's Word, our souls step out from the canopy of God's protective presence. Our defenses are down and our armor is removed. In other words, our minds and our hearts become filled with anxiety because our focus is not on God's Truth, which is final, but the trials of life which are always shifting and ever changing. Knowing and standing on God's truth is our armor and protection against all of the feelings, anxieties, fears, and worries life throws at us.

- Pray that the promises of God's Word would fill your mind and guard your heart.

- Pray that even in the midst of trials and circumstances, your mind would be calm and your heart would be settled in God's Truth.

- Pray that the angels of God would be encamped around you and your family.

- Pray Ephesians 6, that you would put on the whole armor of God and be protected in every spiritual battle.

Day Seven

HEAVEN'S PERSPECTIVE

DAILY PERSONAL TRANSFORMATION

MORNING | ETERNAL TREASURES

Scripture

> *Do not lay up for yourselves treasures on earth, where moth and rust destroy and where thieves break in and steal; but lay up for yourselves treasures in heaven, where neither moth nor rust destroys and where thieves do not break in and steal. For where your treasure is, there your heart will be also* (Matthew 6:19-21).

Devotional

Society tells us that having more stuff on earth will make us happy. The message we get is: "Work harder so you can make more money and buy a beautiful home, a better vehicle, and a nicer wardrobe." That's not to say that Christians should live in squalid conditions and look like they are barely making ends meet, but we should have an eternal perspective on possessions. This will play out in how we spend the resources God has entrusted to us. Everything we own, even the things we worked to buy, are a result of God's grace toward us, because He gives us the ability to earn income (see Deut. 8:17-18). The reason that God blesses us is so that we can be a blessing to others.

Laying up treasures in Heaven doesn't solely pertain to giving finances away; it pertains to the way we spend our time, talents, and energy as well. God has given each of us gifts, and we get to choose how we spend those gifts. In order to spend them wisely today, we need an eternal perspective.

Prayer Journal

What are the things you value most in life? What gives you a sense of fulfillment? Talk to God about where your priorities are, and ask Him if anything needs readjusting.

Consider what percentage of your resources (money, time, talents, and energy) are being used to bless people. Dialogue with God about this as well.

_____

_____

_____

_____

_____

_____

AFTERNOON | TRUST AND SEEK GOD

Scripture

> *Therefore I say to you, do not worry about your life, what you will eat or what you will drink; nor about your body, what you will put on. Is not life more than food and the body more than clothing? ...But seek first the kingdom of God and His righteousness, and all these things shall be added to you (Matthew 6:25,33).*

Devotional

It can be easy to become wrapped up in the daily things of life, so much so that you become anxious about them. But when you focus on the things

God has for you to do and keep your focus on who He is and His faithfulness toward you, your anxiety will melt away and you will realize God takes care of all your needs. You can trust that your heavenly Father will provide what you need in every area of life because He loves you so much!

Prayer Journal

What things have you been able to hand over to God and trust that He is taking care of them? Have you noticed freedom from anxiety during this fast? Or have you noticed things you might be holding on to tightly? If you have noticed that you have too tight of a grip on some things, pray and surrender them to your heavenly Father's care.

Take a moment to consider the daily things God provides for you, and thank Him for them.

_____

_____

_____

_____

_____

_____

EVENING | SEEING CLEARLY FROM HEAVEN'S PERSPECTIVE

Scripture

> Do not judge, or you too will be judged. For in the same way you judge others, you will be judged, and with the measure you use, it will be measured to you (Matthew 7:1-2 NIV).

Devotional

Jesus didn't come to condemn the world. He came to save it! It is not our job to judge people. It is our job to love them.

What if the person genuinely has visible sin in his or her life and claims to be a believer in Jesus? First, ask God if there is a "plank" (sin) in your own life, and take care of that. Then ask God if you should be the one to confront the person living in sin and how you should do that, or if you need to simply pray for them and trust God will work it out with the person. He is big enough to help people take care of their messes without us.

Prayer Journal

Have you found yourself being critical lately? Most of the time what we see in others is a reflection of what is going on inside of us. Inspect yourself and ask the Holy Spirit if there is something in you (it could be a lie you believe) that is skewing your perspective. Then ask what the truth is.

Pray and ask God to give you Heaven's perspective and the ability to love people around you with His love. He may give you an entirely new perspective on why people act the way they do.

Pray for an increase of compassion for people and a heart to restore and not condemn.

Thank God for the grace and forgiveness He has freely given to you.

_____

_____

_____

_____

_____

_____

_____

Day Eight

GOD'S WILL

CORPORATE PRAYER DIRECTIVE

Your kingdom come. Your will be done on earth as it is in heaven (Matthew 6:10).

God's will is not as mysterious as some make it out to be. In the end, it involves us looking at a pretty specific blueprint and representing it through our lives and churches. The blueprint is *on earth as it is in heaven*. God's will is for everything down here to come into agreement with how everything looks up there, in heaven. Even though we will not see the fullness of this come to pass this side of eternity, we must press in to experience every good thing Jesus made available to us released into our sphere of influence. Before we seek God's specific assignment for our individual lives, it is important for us to understand what His *ultimate agenda* is for humanity. There are many areas where His Kingdom can effect change and bring transformation. However, the starting place is the redeemed spirit. Remember, Jesus told us that the Kingdom of God is within us (see Luke 17:21). The first place His Kingdom comes is into the human spirit—when someone gives his or her heart to Jesus Christ. From then, that person begins a lifestyle of transformation. They were transformed at salvation and are continually being transformed as the Kingdom of God becomes their new way of life. This is our first assignment and God's perfect will: *Introducing people to His Kingdom.*

- Pray that the Holy Spirit gives you practical, everyday ideas and strategies on how to share the love and message of Jesus with people in your life.

- Pray for boldness to take advantage of God-ordained opportunities to demonstrate the love and power of Jesus to people (through encouragement, prayer, sharing your testimony, healing, etc.).

- Pray for the Lord to give you specific names of people He wants you to minister to, and ask the Holy Spirit *how* He wants you to minister to them.

- Pray that you would not be so busy that you miss out on everyday opportunities to advance God's Kingdom.

Day Eight

REAL RELATIONSHIP

DAILY PERSONAL TRANSFORMATION

MORNING | ACCESS THROUGH RELATIONSHIP

Scripture

Ask, and it will be given to you; seek, and you will find; knock, and it will be opened to you. For everyone who asks receives, and he who seeks finds, and to him who knocks it will be opened (Matthew 7:7-8).

Devotional

When we have a good friendship with someone, we know that we can feel free to initiate contact with them and ask them for help in our time of need. We don't hesitate to call or text them when we have an urgent prayer request or when we are feeling lonely and just want to talk. Similarly, when we have a real relationship with our Heavenly Father (made possible by believing in His son Jesus and receiving His forgiveness), we can feel free to initiate contact with Him to talk and ask for help in our time of need. He is not far away and it is His joy to answer our requests and commune with us. We have access to Him and all of Heaven's provision through our relationship.

Prayer Journal

Have you felt hesitancy in approaching God to talk to Him or ask Him for help? How do you see God the Father? Is He approachable or distant? If He is distant, ask Him to reveal His true nature to you (it might be a mental picture, a sense, or a word from Him). Write down what He says.

Write down some things you are asking God for, whether it be for yourself, your friends, or your family. Expect God to answer your requests, as they are in agreement with His Word.

_____

_____

_____

_____

_____

_____

_____

AFTERNOON | THE NARROW WAY

Scripture

> *Enter through the narrow gate; for the gate is wide and the way is broad that leads to destruction, and there are many who enter through it. For the gate is small and the way is narrow that leads to life, and there are few who find it* (Matthew 7:13-14 NASB).

Devotional

The meaning of this passage is that by believing Jesus is Lord, that He came to die on the cross to take away our sins, we enter the "narrow gate" into a real relationship with God the Father. This is not normally the popular thing to do, but it is the *only* way that leads to eternal life with God.

By choosing to live a healthy lifestyle, we are choosing the narrow way that leads to life and health. Jesus came to give us life and life abundantly (see John 10:10). He wants us to live life to the full! We get to choose how to handle the resources He entrusts to us, including our bodies, and the choices we make will affect the quality of our life. The quality of our life and health will affect every arena of the spheres of influence we have. It might not be easy to make healthy lifestyle choices, but the effect will certainly impact our life and the lives of those surrounding us.

Prayer Journal

Thank the Lord for saving you and showing you the narrow gate to salvation and narrow way to good health. Ask the Lord for ways you can stay spiritually and physically healthy once the fast is finished.

_____

_____

_____

_____

_____

_____

_____

EVENING | RELATIONSHIP IS THE MOST IMPORTANT THING

Scripture

Not everyone who says to me, "Lord, Lord," will enter the kingdom of heaven, but only the one who does the will of my Father who is in heaven. Many will say to me on that day, "Lord, Lord, did we not prophesy in your name and in your name drive out demons and in your name perform many miracles?" Then I will tell them plainly, "I never knew you. Away from me, you evildoers!" (Matthew 7:21-23 NIV)

Devotional

This is kind of a scary passage because we would assume that people who are doing signs and wonders in Jesus' name would certainly enter the Kingdom of Heaven. But it is possible that Jesus will say to them, "I never knew you." That indicates that they did not have an authentic relationship with God through Jesus.

It is not about what you do for God or what miracles God does through you. It is all about having a relationship with God. Take time to develop it daily.

Prayer Journal

Spend some time telling God how much you love Him and let Him tell you how much He loves you. Try doing this once or twice a day, when you wake up in the morning and right before you go to sleep.

_____

_____

_____

_____

_____

_____

_____

Day Nine

GOD'S VISION

CORPORATE PRAYER DIRECTIVE

Where there is no vision, the people perish... (Proverbs 29:18 KJV).

We recognize that there is a world to save, and in order for the world to be transformed, we need to be in sync with what God is doing *in our lives*. Saving the world sounds like a daunting task, but the truth is, we participate in God's great redemptive plan every day of our lives when we fulfill the assignment He has given each one of us. This is why it is so important to pray for vision. Specific vision. Maybe you have already received a specific vision from God, or you have received some clarity on your life purpose from God. Ask for this to be clarified and for greater wisdom to be released in how to execute the vision. If you need vision, this is a great time to ask for it. The key is discerning what the Holy Spirit wants done in this unique hour and moving forward on that vision with focus and intentionality.

- Pray for the Lord to refresh your sense of personal vision—what He has uniquely called you to do in this specific season of your life.

- Ask the Lord to help you plan for the future: 5, 10, and even 20 years away.

- Pray for the Holy Spirit to give you discernment to focus on the things you are supposed to be focused on and to not be distracted by other things.

- Pray for a greater understanding of what God has called you to do through the gifts and talents He has created you with.

- Pray that you would receive fresh insight on the talents, gifts, and abilities God has given you to advance His Kingdom and fulfill His purpose for your life.

Day Nine

UNSEEN REALITY

Daily Personal Transformation

Morning | Shining for Jesus

Scripture

You are the light of the world. A town built on a hill cannot be hidden. Neither do people light a lamp and put it under a bowl. Instead they put it on its stand, and it gives light to everyone in the house. In the same way, let your light shine before others, that they may see your good deeds and glorify your Father in heaven (Matthew 5:14-16 NIV).

Devotional

When you became a child of God through faith in Jesus Christ, you were rescued from the dominion of darkness into the Kingdom of light (see Col. 1:10-14). You emanate a light that comes from Heaven. The spiritually discerning may sometimes tell you this, but whether or not people see an actual light coming from you, they should notice the good deeds you do and the good attitude you have.

The wonderful thing about shining for Jesus is that you don't have to consciously do it. It is a result of worshiping, meditating on the Word, praying, and focusing on God's face and His love for you. So don't be surprised if someone tells you that you are glowing! Tell them about the fast you've been on, but also give glory to God by sharing about the spiritual side of your journey toward good health as well.

Prayer Journal

What do you think it looks like to "shine for Jesus?"

_____

_____

_____

_____

_____

_____

_____

AFTERNOON | THE ARMOR OF GOD

Scripture

Finally, be strong in the Lord and in his mighty power. Put on the full armor of God, so that you can take your stand against the devil's schemes (Ephesians 6:10-11 NIV).

Devotional

There is an unseen battle going on around us. Maybe you have been feeling opposition these past nine days. It could be just your body responding, but it could also be from the enemy. If you've been hearing negative thoughts in your mind, don't assume that they are your own thoughts. They may very well be from the enemy because he can put thoughts in your mind that sound like your own.

Ephesians 6 tells us how to dress spiritually to stand against the devil's schemes. A good exercise is to put on the armor of God in the morning as you dress as a prophetic statement of being spiritually prepared for battle. God has given us everything we need to stand and engage in battle and win!

Prayer Journal

Open up your Bible to Ephesians 6. What does it look like for you to be clothed in the armor of God?

Thank God for the armor and weapons He has given you to stand strong and win spiritual battles.

_____

_____

_____

_____

_____

_____

_____

EVENING | BELIEVE AND RECEIVE

Scripture

Now faith is the substance of things hoped for, the evidence of things not seen (Hebrews 11:1).

Devotional

There is an unseen world of heavenly provision waiting to be accessed. Faith is the currency by which we can access heavenly provision. All we have to do is believe and receive, just like when we believed in Jesus' payment for our sins and received the free gift of salvation. Have faith and believe that God is good and that He will give you what you pray for (if it is His best for you) even though circumstances may look totally different. Don't look at what is seen, but what is unseen (see 2 Cor. 4:18).

Prayer Journal

You have been asking God for many over the course of this fast. Imagine the Father giving you your heart's desire and yourself receiving that gift. Thank Him for the answers to your prayers that are coming.

_____

_____

_____

_____

_____

_____

Day Ten

THANKSGIVING FOR WHAT GOD IS GOING TO DO

CORPORATE PRAYER DIRECTIVE

Be anxious for nothing, but in everything by prayer and supplication, with thanksgiving, let your requests be made known to God (Philippians 4:6).

We've invested this past ten days in prayer and fasting. I know it has been difficult on our flesh, but I am expecting that many, if not all of you, have experienced a transformational time in your relationship with God. Even if you think, "I don't feel anything," I encourage you—the Holy Spirit is not finished yet! We need to live in a place of expectant thanksgiving. Fasting is sowing into supernatural soil. We may not see how it all works right up front, but we can have hearts full of thanksgiving and praise, knowing that God is working behind the scenes, getting ready to release breakthrough, miracles, and new levels of relationship with Him in the days ahead!

- Praise God for the spiritual transformation that is taking place in your life!

- Deeper intimacy with God

- More effective prayer

- Renewed purpose and vision

- Victory over sinful habits

- Praise God for the physical transformation that is taking place in your life!

- Weight loss

- New, healthy eating habits

- Commitment to diet and exercise

- Fresh awareness that your body is God's temple

- Praise God for the emotional transformation that is taking place in your life!

- Peace instead of anxiety, worry, and fear

- Joy instead of depression

- Freedom from destructive emotions

- Mind cleared of negative thoughts

Day Ten

GOD'S HIGHER ROAD

DAILY PERSONAL TRANSFORMATION

MORNING | TAKE THE HIGH ROAD

Scripture

> *You have heard that it was said, "Eye for eye, and tooth for tooth."
> But I tell you, do not resist an evil person. If anyone slaps you
> on the right cheek, turn to them the other cheek also* (Matthew
> 5:38-39 NIV).

Devotional

The natural reaction to being hurt by people is to hurt them back and protect ourselves from being hurt again. This is when listening to God instead of our feelings needs to come into play. Let's say someone takes advantage of you financially. God may be asking you to bless the person instead of getting back what they owe you. This makes no sense in our minds, but we only see part of the puzzle. God sees all of the factors, plus He sees into the future. Your action of kindness and generosity could break down their resistance to God's love.

Or let's say someone slanders you behind your back. Your first reaction will be to defend yourself, but God might be telling you to be quiet. Do you trust that God is big enough to defend you without you speaking out?

It may not be easy, but we can ask the Holy Spirit to help us take the high road, and we will be promoted spiritually for obeying.

Prayer Journal

Ask God how you can apply this principle to your life right now or in the future and write down what He says.

_____

_____

_____

_____

_____

_____

_____

AFTERNOON | LOVE YOUR ENEMIES

Scripture

> You're familiar with the old written law, "Love your friend," and its unwritten companion, "Hate your enemy." I'm challenging that. I'm telling you to love your enemies. Let them bring out the best in you, not the worst. When someone gives you a hard time, respond with the energies of prayer, for then you are working out of your true selves, your God-created selves (Matthew 5:43-45 MSG).

Devotional

Beyond not retaliating when we are hurt, God actually wants us to love people who hurt us. He also wants us to love people who have different agendas and viewpoints from us. How is this possible? It is only possible by the power of the Holy Spirit who lives inside of us. He gives us the ability to love people, no matter how they treat us. Loving our enemies may not come naturally, however, so it is our decision whether or not we will enlist God's help to take His higher road and love every person with His love.

Prayer Journal

Think of someone who has hurt you. Ask the Holy Spirit for grace to love them with God's love and forgive them if you haven't already. Write down a prayer for them.

_____

_____

_____

_____

_____

_____

_____

EVENING | GOD'S DREAMS FOR US

Scripture

Now to him who is able to do immeasurably more than all we ask or imagine, according to his power that is at work within us (Ephesians 3:20 NIV).

Devotional

God is able to do more than all we could ask or imagine! Isn't that incredible? Our heavenly Father has better plans for us than our earthly parents could have ever dreamed, and He has the power to enable us to fulfill the destiny He has for us. His ideas and dreams for our lives are even better than our own.

As you are finishing this fast, press into discovering the dreams that God has for your life. They are so good because He is so good and He loves you so much!

Prayer Journal

Take some time to dream and vision cast with God. What are things you want to see happen in this world in your lifetime? What role could you play in bringing God's Kingdom to to pass? Ask God for practical steps you can take to make these dreams a reality.

_____

_____

_____

_____

_____

_____

_____

Appendix A

BENEFITS OF FASTING

Spiritual Benefits of Fasting

1. Fasting can bring you closer to God.

2. Fasting can make you more sensitive to God's voice.

3. Fasting helps break addictions.

4. Fasting shows us our weakness and allows us to rely on God's strength.

E.E. Puriton wrote in his book, *Philosophy of Fasting*, "There is not a habit or weakness that can survive a siege of prayer and fasting. Prayer alone is just one-half of the battle."

Emotional Benefits of Fasting

1. Fasting helps support healthy emotions.

2. Fasting clears your mind of negative thoughts.

3. Fasting can bring peace.

Dr. Otto F.H. Buchinger, who supervised more than 70,000 fasts, states, "Fasting is...a royal road to health for anyone who agrees to take it for the transformation of the body, mind and spirit."

12 Physical Benefits of Fasting

> Paracelcus, famed 15th-century physician and alchemist who believed in the body's ability to heal itself, says fasting activates "The Healer Within."

1. Fasting helps break addictions to junk food, drinking, and smoking.

2. Fasting supports the body's detoxification systems.

3. Fasting promotes healthy weight loss.

4. Fasting promotes healthy energy levels.

5. Fasting supports healthy aging, healthy skin, and a glowing complexion.

6. Fasting promotes healthy memory, focus, and concentration.

7. Fasting reduces stress and promotes sound sleep.

8. Fasting supports cardiovascular health.

9. Fasting promotes healthy digestion and elimination.

10. Fasting supports healthy inflammation response and promotes joint comfort.

11. Fasting supports healthy immune system function.

12. Fasting promotes healthy hormonal balance.

Appendix B

PRAYER FOR BLESSING

Today I pray that, like Job, God would surround you with a hedge of protection and that you would have twice the blessings in the latter part of your life from this day forward.

I pray that, like Abraham, you would grow wealthy with cattle, gold, and silver.

That like Isaac, you'd plant a field and reap a hundred-fold harvest.

That like Jacob, with wisdom and discernment you would grow your flocks and herds.

That like Joseph, the dream that God's given you will be salvation to many.

That like Moses, the Lord will reveal Himself to you and show you His glory.

That like Bazalel, who helped build the tabernacle, the Lord would anoint you for the specific task that He's called you to accomplish.

That like Joshua, God will fill you with the spirit of wisdom.

That like the Children of Israel, you'd live in lands that you didn't buy, with barns and houses that you didn't build filled with things that you didn't purchase, drinking from wells and springs that you didn't know existed and eating from vineyards and groves that you didn't plant. That He'd care for your land and water it, and enrich it abundantly. That He'd bless the fruit of your trees, the crops of your land, the grass of your fields, and the calves of your herds. That He'd bring the spring and autumn rains, softening the land with showers, that your threshing floors will be filled with grain; your vats will overflow with new wine and oil, that your bulls will never fail to breed and your cows will never miscarry, that there would be none sick among you and none barren, that you would smite a thousand enemies as the Lord fights for you and you would return from battle with silver, gold, bronze, iron, and clothing. That your sons in their youth will be like well-nurtured plants, and your daughters will be like pillars carved to adorn a palace. That your sheep will increase by thousands, by tens of thousands in your fields.

That as you bring the tithe into the storehouse, the Lord will throw open the floodgates of heaven and pour out so much blessing that you will not have enough room for it. That He will prevent pests from devouring your crops, and the vines in your fields will not cast their fruit. Then all the nations will call you blessed, for yours will be a delightful land.

That like David, God would give you a blueprint of what He would like you to build for Him.

That like Solomon, He would give you a wise and understanding heart.

That like Uzziah, there would be good men caring for your cattle in the foothills and that you'd have a love and understanding of the soil.

That like Daniel, God would give you ten times the wisdom, favor, understanding, and discernment of all those who don't know Him.

And that like Peter, you'd cast your net on the right side of the boat and catch 153 fish.

Not by power, not by might, but by Your Spirit, O God.

This is my prayer for you.

Appendix C

PRAYER FOR HEALING

Note: This prayer is specifically written for cancer, but wherever you note the specific disease name, change it out and replace it with whatever health challenge you are currently facing (diabetes, anxiety, multiple sclerosis, IBS, etc.) and the body part it effects.

Every organ and tissue of my body functions in the perfection that God created it to function. I forbid any malfunction in my body in Jesus' name.

The same Spirit that raised Jesus from the dead dwells in me, permeating His life through my veins, sending healing throughout my body.

The spirit and life of God's Word flows in me cleansing my blood of every disease and impurity.

My immune system grows stronger day by day. I speak life to my immune system. I forbid confusion in my immune system.

"Lymph glands, you are healed in Jesus' name; I command you to be normal in size and to function normally as my God created you to function." No weapon formed against me shall prosper. Because the Lord is for me, no disease can be against me.

Every cell that does not promote life and health in my body is cut off from its life source. My immune system will not allow tumorous growth to live in my body in Jesus' name.

That which God has not planted is dissolved and rooted out of my body in the name of Jesus. First Peter 2:24 is engrafted into every fiber of my being, and I am alive with the life of God.

Jesus bore the curse for me, therefore, I forbid growths and tumors to inhabit my body. The life of God within me dissolves growths and tumors, and my strength and health is restored.

Growths and tumors have no right to my body. They are a thing of the past, for I am delivered from the authority of darkness. In Jesus Name!

The law of the Spirit of Life in Christ Jesus has made me free from the law of sin and death, therefore I will not allow sin, sickness, or death to lord it over me.

I will not allow the devil any inroad to attempt to steal, kill, and destroy me. The Bible says that I have already been healed; I am more than a conqueror; I am an overcomer—the head and not the tail; I am above only and not beneath; He wishes above all things that my soul prosper and that I would be in good health. These are not just words; these are God's promises to me. He loves me; He wants me to be victorious on earth as it is in heaven.

I have set a boundary around my family with a blood line that is the blood of our Messiah. No weapon formed against me can cross this bloodline that is surrounding me! No defeated demon from the pit of Hell can affect me or harm me. Even though I walk through the valley of the shadow of death, I will not fear! Satan, you have no authority here and must get out of my life and out of my body because I have been redeemed by the blood of the Lamb. I have been translated from the powers of darkness and translated into God's Kingdom! I am healed and nothing, and I mean nothing can or will come against me. Only what God has planted in my body will be in my body, and remain there. Anything that God has not planted is rooted out of my body, in the name of Jesus. I have had it with the enemy and his attacks. I stand on the word of God and trust Him fully; only He can bring me through these circumstances victoriously. Only Him! No food, medicine, or man-made thing can do what my Savior has already done and will continue to do for me. I will trust in God, because He loves me.

I don't have to bow down to the name "cancer." Cancer has to bow down to me, because God's spirit indwells me and I have become a joint heir with Jesus as the Righteousness of Christ. He says in His word that He has given me power to tread on serpents and trample on our enemy. The devil is defeated, and God has given me victory when He shed His blood on the tree. God's Word is sharper than any two-edged sword and better able to heal than any surgeon's blade. God's promises are true and better able to cure than any physician's medicines. I am a healed man, a healed woman. It has already been done for me. Amen!

Appendix D

EA PULSE INGREDIENTS

EA Pulse Antioxidant Fruits
Sprouted Seed Clusters (Sunflower Seed,* Coconut (flakes),* Flaxseed,* Chia Seed,* Hemp Seed,* Pumpkin Seed,* Sesame Seed,* Banana,* Date,* Fig,* Mulberry,* Black Sesame Seed*), Superfruit Blend (Goji,* Strawberry,* Raspberry,* Blackberry,* Pomegranate,* Raisin,* Cherry,* Currant,* Cranberry* (sweetened w/Apple Juice), Acai,* Noni,* Mangosteen,* Plum,* Red Apple,* Pink Grapefruit*), Sprouted Nut Blend (Pecan,* Almond,* Cashew,* Walnut*), Terrain Living Herbal Infusion (Fermented Ginger,* Fermented Echinacea,* Fermented Lavender,* Fermented Milk Thistle,* Fermented Cinnamon,* Fermented Rooibos,* and Fermented Ginseng* in a base of live probiotics and enzymes)

EA Pulse Omega Fruits
Sprouted Seed Clusters (Sunflower Seed,* Coconut (flakes),* Flaxseed,* Chia Seed,* Hemp Seed,* Pumpkin Seed,* Sesame Seed,* Banana,* Date,* Fig,* Mulberry,* Black Sesame Seed*), Superfruit Blend (Pineapple,* Mango,* Golden Raisin,* Wild Mountain Apricot,* Peach,* Sea Buckthorn,* Green Apple,* Yellow Grapefruit,* Lemon,* Lime,* Orange,* Tangerine,* Papaya,* Kiwi,* Sprouted Nut Blend (Pecan,* Almond,* Cashew* Walnut*), Terrain Living Herbal Infusion (Fermented Ginger,* Fermented Turmeric,* Fermented Star Anise,* Fermented Lemongrass,* Fermented Black Tea,* Fermented Green Tea,* Fermented Holy Basil,* Fermented Oregano, and Fermented Peppermint in a base of live probiotics and enzymes)

EA Pulse Super Veggies

Sprouted Seed Clusters (Sunflower Seed,* Coconut (flakes),* Flaxseed,* Chia Seed,* Hemp Seed,* Pumpkin Seed,* Sesame Seed,* Onion,* Portabello Mushroom,* Black Sesame Seed*), Super Veggie Blend (Green Pea,* Corn,* Kale,* Green Pepper,* Green Onion,* Broccoli,* Celery,* Collard,* Green Cabbage,* Green Bean,* Cucumber,* Spinach,* Zucchini,* Lettuce,* Brussels Sprouts,* Asparagus,* Purple Onion,* Purple Cabbage,* Beetroot*), Yellow Squash,* Carrot,* Red Pepper,* Tomato,* Butternut Squash,* Yellow Pepper,* Pumpkin,* Sweet Potato,* Radish*), Sprouted Nut Blend (Pecan,* Almond,* Cashew,* Walnut*), Terrain Living Herbal Infusion (Fermented Garlic,* Fermented Turmeric,* Fermented Star Anise,* Fermented Lemongrass,* Fermented Cinnamon,* Fermented Rooibos,* Fermented Ginseng,* Fermented Black Tea,* Fermented Green Tea,* Fermented Holy Basil,* Fermented Oregano,* Fermented Peppermint,* Fermented Echinacea,* Fermented Lavender,* and Fermented Milk Thistle* in a base of live probiotics and enzymes)

*organic

Please note that I encourage you to refrain from any other foods, beverages, or other commonly consumed items during this ten-day period. This includes but is not limited to coffee, energy drinks, gum, mints, or candy.

If you are on medication and/or under the care of a physician, please consult him or her before beginning this or any diet regimen, *and by no means* should you alter your medication dosage or schedule. Please check the ingredients for each of the EA Pulse products, and do not undertake the 10-Day Daniel Diet if you have known allergies to any of the ingredients.

ABOUT JORDAN RUBIN

Known as America's Biblical Health Coach, Jordan Rubin is the *New York Times* best-selling author of *The Maker's Diet* and twenty additional health titles, including his recent book, *Live Beyond Organic*. An international motivational speaker and host of the weekly television show "Living Beyond Organic," which reaches over 30 million households worldwide, Jordan has lectured on natural health on five continents and 46 states in the U.S.

Jordan Rubin is the founder of Garden of Life, a leading whole food nutritional supplement company, and has earned doctorate degrees in naturopathic medicine, nutrition, and natural therapies. In 2009, he fulfilled a lifelong dream by starting Beyond Organic, a vertically integrated company specializing in organic foods, beverages, and skin and body care products that includes farming operations on over 8,000 organic acres in Missouri and Georgia.

Jordan resides in southern Missouri with his wife, Nicki, and their three children, Joshua, Samuel, and Alexis.